Cilantro Essential Oils

Benefits, Properties, Applications, Studies & Recipes

by Ann Sullivan

Published in USA by:

Ann Sullivan
217 N. Seacrest Blvd #9
Boynton Beach
FL 33425

© Copyright 2015

I ISBN-13: 978-1544738970
ISBN-10: 1544738978

Table of Contents

Introduction

What are essential oils and how might they be used for therapeutic purposes?

Essential oils are ultra-potent oils extracted from plants and flowers that have been utilized in medicine for centuries. Presently, they are most commonly used to supplement pharmaceutical medication, but they can also be an effective alternative to pharmaceuticals in the event that there is no access to them. Before dismissing essential oils as a means to support the body's natural defenses against injury and illness, take a look at the historical evidence of the oils' medicinal competence in practice. The average age-old medical text will demonstrate that essential oils, herbs, and plenty of other natural ingredients have, for thousands of years, successfully enhanced immune function to meet and defeat any number of ailments and injuries. Though traditional medicine is considered "alternative" now, it was once the gold standard. Perhaps it still should be, as these natural age-tested remedies can fortify the body's defenses against everything from simple maladies, like headaches, cuts, and bruises to serious diseases, like cancer.

Essential oils are deemed "essential," because the oils are composed of the "essence" of the plant. The difference between essential oils and other oils – like olive oil or vegetable oil, for instance – is that essential oils have high volatility and reduced fixation, which results in faster evaporation, enabling their popular use in aromatherapy. Even at high temperatures, olive and vegetable oils do not evaporate.

Essential oils are especially necessary when it comes to a major natural or man-made disaster or potential viral outbreak. In these dire situations, people may not have quick access to their standard pharmaceutical supply; so essential oils, along with other alternative medicines, will be the go-to health aids in the case of social collapse, viral outbreak, or devastating natural disaster. When medical access is unavailable, alternatives to our modern-day standard are the only chance we have to keep pathogens at bay.

Most people do not realize that they already use essential oils every day. They are in perfumes, shampoos, soaps, and ointments; they are even used in furniture polish. Why are they found in so many aromatic products? Well, because essential oils are super concentrated aromatic liquids, so their scent is remarkably strong. Let us put this into perspective: to steam tea, use a few leaves of peppermint or juniper; to produce a single ounce of essential oil, five whole *pounds* of peppermint or juniper leaves are required. Some sources claim that to produce twelve pounds of essential oil would necessitate an acre of peppermint, juniper, or any other oil being produced en masse. Unlike vegetable oil, you do not often find concentrated therapeutic-grade essential oils sold in bulk; instead the oils are often sold in easily carried small, dark bottles, perfect for the GOOD bag (Get Out Of Dodge). That is exactly what this book is aiming to help people plan for – getting out of dodge with the most vital of essential oils intact, in particular a good supply of Cilantro essential oil.

Why Cilantro, you ask? Well, in order to get quickly up to speed on this most essential of oils, below we have provided a condensed synopsis of Cilantro, after which we will outline in greater detail the oil's history, properties, and common therapeutic uses, so that you – the consumer – might have a better understanding of the oil's benefits and applications. We have even provided supportive remedies for pure Cilantro, as well as blended recipes that incorporate the valuable oil. Chapter 3 will further detail past scientific research on Cilantro essential oil.

Now, let's get down to it – **Essential Oil 101: The Basics of Cilantro**

Origin: Cilantro, or Coriandrum sativum, originated in Hungary and has been used for hundreds of years to flavor culinary dishes, as well as to aid digestion. The Chinese have been promoting Cilantro's medicinal properties for centuries.

Coriander and Cilantro are often used synonymously, but they are actually extracted from different parts of the same parsley plant; coriander from the seeds and Cilantro from the leaves.

Description: Cilantro oil is commonly extracted

through steam distillation. The leaves are most often used. The oil is yellow in color, thin in consistency, and has a medium sharp herb scent.

Uses: Beyond those applications previously mentioned, additional uses for Cilantro essential oil include supporting the body's natural function against indigestion, arthritis, colic, exhaustion, flu, migraines, nausea, colds, diarrhea, flatulence, muscle pain, and rheumatism. Its antioxidant properties also help leach heavy metals from the body.

Properties: Antioxidant, analgesic, antibacterial, antifungal, anti-inflammatory, anti-rheumatic, antispasmodic, antidepressant, sedative, carminative, stomachic, digestive, and stimulant.

Application: Dilute 1:1 with a carrier oil. Apply topically, inhale directly, diffuse, or use as a dietary supplement.

Safety Precautions: Cilantro has been approved by the FDA for internal consumption and can be used as a dietary supplement. Do not use excessively.

Fun facts: The fresh leaves of Cilantro are utilized in many international cuisines, including in Chinese, Thai, Indian, Mexican, and Russian dishes. In Mexico, Cilantro is used in the making of guacamole and salsa. In India, it is used in salads, chutneys, and as a garnish alongside dal. In Russia, Cilantro is used in salads.

Chapter 1:
Benefits of Cilantro Essential Oil

Cilantro oil offers a number of therapeutic benefits; you may be wondering what these benefits are? In this chapter we will take a closer look at the history of Cilantro and its many uses.

Cultivation of Cilantro

Known as "coriander leaves," "fresh coriander," "dhania," or "Chinese parsley," Cilantro comes from the Apiaceae family of annual herbs. The plant grows across a wide range of regions, from southwest Asia to northern Africa and southern Europe. The plant grows to be 20" tall, with leaves in various shapes growing broad at the base and thin at the height of the plant, where the white or pale pink flowers sprout. The fruit of this plant is cylindrical and may be eaten, but more often, the seeds are added to other foods as a spice.

A History of Cilantro

The word "coriander" essentially derives from the ancient Mycenaean Greek "ford koriadnon," which is similar in spelling to the name of Ariadne, Minos' daughter. Because of the herb's ubiquitous use in Mexican cuisine, the most common word used for the herb in North America is Cilantro, which is the Spanish word for coriander. The entire plant is edible and both Cilantro and coriander are used in a number of other international cuisines, including African, Latin American, Portuguese, Brazilian, Middle Eastern, Tex-Mex, Asian, Chinese, Scandinavian, Caucasian, and Mediterranean. The phytochemicals in coriander are also known help prevent food spoilage.

The seeds of the plant have a distinctly different aroma and taste than the leaves. Cilantro tends to possess a citrusy note, although some consider the aroma pungent with a particularly unpleasant soapy overtone to the taste of the leaves. However, as mentioned, the use of Cilantro leaves is common in all types of cuisine; the herb is frequently added to the dish raw, and directly before serving, instead of cooked, as cooking reduces the flavor of Cilantro, as does freezing and drying. In Central Asia and India, Cilantro is often cooked in large amounts until the flavor is slightly reduced.

The leaves and seeds of this plant also provide

different nutritional content. The seeds, for instance, offer calcium, iron, selenium, magnesium, fiber, and manganese, while the leaves are much higher in vitamin and mineral content, especially vitamins A, C, and K.

The historical roots of the plant are debatable. Growing in the wild across such an expansive region, stretching from southern Europe across the Near East, pinpointing the plant's beginnings is difficult at best. However, one of the oldest archaeological discoveries of coriander was in the Nahal Hemar Cave in Israel, where it was found alongside Neolithic Pre-Pottery era. Another of the oldest finds was in the tomb of Tutankhamen, where half a liter of coriander was discovered. The plant is believed to have been cultivated in ancient Egypt, as it does not grow wild there. Similarly, ancient Greece is believed to have cultivated the plant since the second millennium BC, where according to the Pylos' Linear B tablets, the plant's oils served perfumery, while its seeds and leaves served as a spice and an herb, respectively. Transported to North America by the British in 1670, coriander was among the first plants to be cultivated by the early British colonists.

Chemical Components

In order to generate the essential oil from Cilantro the leaves must be steam distilled. This results in the oil's key chemical components, which are primarily linalool, borneol, cineole, dipentene, cymene, terpinolene, terpineol, phellandrene, and pinene. Cilantro leaves and stems also provide polyphenolic flavonoids, which are rich in antioxidants. These include apigenin, quercetin, rhamnetin, and kaempferol.

Main Properties of Cilantro Essential Oil

Along with the properties previously mentioned in the introduction, Cilantro oil possesses antioxidant, analgesic, antibacterial, antifungal, anti-inflammatory, anti-rheumatic, antispasmodic, antidepressant, sedative, carminative, stomachic, digestive, and stimulant properties. With such a versatile range, Cilantro is well equipped to fight off any pathogen in the body.

Cilantro, as mentioned, is composed of linalool, borneol, cineole, dipentene, cymene, terpinolene, terpineol, phellandrene, and pinene. These components are what instill the enormously beneficial properties within Cilantro essential oil. We will outline these properties below.

Antioxidant

Anything high in antioxidants – whether fruit, beans, or essential oils – is a powerful advocate for the body. Antioxidants both protect against free radicals and repair damage. What are free radicals? Free radicals are destructive chemicals that invade the body, produced by substances both inside and out. Some free radicals (or oxidants) form through normal bodily reactions, like inflammation, metabolism, and aerobic respiration. Other free radicals form outside the body, but enter it due to exposure. These include harmful pollutants, toxins, smoking, drinking alcohol, X-rays, and UV rays, to name a few. Although our bodies produce their own antioxidants, these often become damaged as we grow older; thus, introducing antioxidants into our bodies via essential oils allows these nutrients and enzymes to assist in chemical reactions which destroy the oxidants, or free radicals. Cilantro essential oil is a moderate antioxidant, aiming to detox the body of free radicals that lead to disease

Analgesic

Cilantro's analgesic qualities make it an effective supplement for pain relief to be used in supporting relief from headache, sprains, injuries, wounds, scars, bruises, burns, and arthritis. It is a surefire aid to any sports muscle sprain, or recovery pain from surgery.

Antibacterial

Cilantro's antibacterial properties make it a powerful protectant against diseases produced by bacteria, such as oral, digestive, and urinary tract bacterial infection. What is great is that, unlike some prescription drugs, Cilantro has no ill effects on bodily health, or on the healthy natural flora that exists within the stomach and intestines.

Antifungal

While bacteria and viruses are bad enough, fungi commonly lead to the deadliest infections, whether external or internal. The ears, throat, and nose are the most likely to become infected by fungi, the infections of which can be both excruciating and unsightly. If left untreated, fungal infections can kill, as they may spread to the brain. Cilantro essential oil protects against these infections and is particularly effective against skin infections.

Anti-inflammatory

External or internal inflammation can be reduced through the use of Cilantro essential oil. For instance, if a patient has swollen fingers from arthritis or a swollen knee from a sport's injury, oral application of Cilantro essential oil may decrease irritation or redness, while also soothing the pain that accompanies inflammation.

Antispasmodic

The antispasmodic properties of Cilantro oil make it beneficial to such health issues as chronic coughing and other respiratory conditions, along with surgical processes, such as colonoscopy and gastroscopy.

Antidepressant

When it comes to psychological issues, the uplifting scent of Cilantro combats negative thoughts and supports relief from depression.

Sedative

As a sedative, Cilantro sedates and calms by reducing anxiety, excitement, or irritability. Though sedatives alone do not alleviate pain, they do calm the patient, making them less stressed and more compliant.

Carminative

By supporting the reduction of excess gas buildup and/or removal of gas from the intestines, Cilantro essential oil provides relief from abdominal pain, excess sweating, and uncomfortable indigestion.

Stomachic

As a stomachic, Cilantro improves stomach function, boosts appetite, and helps to tone the stomach. The oil helps control the stomach's bile, acid, and gastric liquids.

Digestive

By boosting the production of absorptive enzymes, the digestibility of nutrients, and the secretion of digestive juices, Cilantro essential oil aids the digestive tract significantly, which can have a significant impact on the body's overall health by increasing those nutrients absorbed from food.

Stimulant

Stimulants are often referred to as "uppers." This is because they produce mental and/or physical improvements, or temporary enhancements of your bodily functions. For instance, you may grow more alert and awake, or quicker on your feet after using a stimulant. Cilantro can provide this temporary boost in mental and physical function.

Antirheumatic

Whereas the anti-inflammatory properties that Cilantro possesses support the symptoms of arthritis, they do not necessarily influence the underlying cause. However, Cilantro is also anti-rheumatic, which means it can be used to slow the disease progression of rheumatoid arthritis.

Common Medicinal Uses

With a history rooted in international cuisine, Cilantro was used to support the digestive system by soothing digestive flow. Moreover, the oil's properties promote healthy cardiovascular health and blood pressure, while also supporting psychological strains, like anxiety and depression. Below are a few more ways in which Cilantro can play a role in the body's overall health.

Digestive Aid

A healthy digestive tract means a healthy body, so maintaining good digestion can make a world of difference when it comes to overall wellness. The digestive tract is between 25' – 30' in length. If the length of it is not working properly, then there is a chance that food will get caught up somewhere along the tract and begin to rot within the body. Cilantro effectively supports the digestive tract's natural function by producing digestive juices and enzymes and inducing bile flow throughout the digestive organs. The fiber content of Cilantro helps relieve gastrointestinal issues, such as upset stomach, flatulence, nausea, and indigestion.

Cardiovascular Health

Cardiovascular health can be maintained through the abundance of vitamins and minerals found in Cilantro essential oil, which include calcium, magnesium, potassium, and iron. The oil contains dietary fiber as well, which along with its other contents, helps to reduce bad cholesterol (LDL) and boost good cholesterol (HDL), resulting in better cardiovascular health. The oil's antioxidant properties and its ability to facilitate the dissolution of cholesterol that accumulates in arteries will also support cardiovascular issues, like heart disease or atherosclerosis.

Maintains Healthy Blood Pressure

Brimming with the vitamins and minerals mentioned above, Cilantro is also low in sodium, which is a good thing when it comes to blood pressure. The oil's ability to reduce LDL cholesterol levels, along with its low-sodium/high-potassium balance positively impacts blood pressure and heart rate, as does its manganese and iron content. Iron supports the production of red blood cells, while manganese works as a co-facilitator to the oil's antioxidant enzyme, superoxide dismutase, which is a significant antioxidant defense in almost all living cells with exposure to oxygen.

Supports Anxiety

The scent of Cilantro has been shown to relieve anxiety, soothe emotion, and calm nerves. The natural sedative eases stress, mental fatigue, nervousness, and exhaustion. If stressors have impacted your anxiety levels, you can combat negative emotions or head them off through an essential oil application of Cilantro, whether aroma, therapeutic, ingested, or topical.

Detoxifies Heavy Metals

This herb is a "chelation agent," or a heavy metal detoxifier. It eliminates heavy metals that enter the body through such environmental inlets as the foods we eat, the products we use, the air we breathe, the water we wash with, and other like factors. These heavy metals can cause emotional and mental issues, heart problems, lung or kidney diseases, weakened bones, or even cancer. What Cilantro does to eliminate metals, like mercury for instance, from entering the central nervous system and the brain, is to draw the metals from the fatty tissue and transfer them into the lymph and the bloodstream, where the metals can be safely removed from the body. Thus, Cilantro can reduce the risk of mercury poisoning or toxicity.

Strengthens Hair Health

If you have unhealthy hair or dandruff, Cilantro is just what you need to give your hair's gloss and strength a boost, while eliminating flaky and itchy scalp. As opposed to the harsh, dry, damaging chemicals in dandruff shampoos, Cilantro is a healthy alternative that serves your skin and hair naturally. Cilantro can also combat hair loss by providing your hair with the proteins and vitamins essential to hair growth.

Bone Health

Cilantro is rich in calcium, a mineral that supports bone durability and regrowth, making the oil an effective source when it comes to strengthening bone health. Cilantro can help decelerate the aging process of bones, combating osteoporosis and other degenerative bone conditions. The entire plant is rich in calcium, but Cilantro leaves, particularly so.

Strengthens Eye Health

High in antioxidants, in vitamins A and C, as well as in minerals like phosphorous, Cilantro can protect against macular degeneration and vision conditions. The oil helps reduce the stress placed on our eyes. Cilantro leaves contain beta-carotene, a chemical that can decelerate ocular aging and vision degeneration.

Safety Precautions & Common Applications

Safety

Some adverse effects may evolve when using pure essential oils. Some essential oils should not be used when pregnant for example. Allergic reactions may occur, especially when applied topically. Always administer an allergy test before committing fully to topical application. When used with other medications, essential oils may react negatively. If on any current prescription medications or chronic illness is present, such as high blood pressure, epilepsy, or liver disease, then researching the effects of essential oils against personal medical history will eliminate any potentially problems.

Cilantro has been approved by the FDA for internal consumption and can be used as a dietary supplement. Use sparingly. Apply topically, diffuse, or use as a dietary supplement.

Blends

Oftentimes, essential oils are manufactured as blends of several pure oils. For instance, a Protective Oil Blend is a mix of cinnamon, clove, rosemary, and eucalyptus. This blend can be used to boost the immune system to help support the body's defenses against colds, viruses, and flus. The downside to blends is that the more oils added to the mix, the higher the probability a patient may react negatively to the blend if he/she is prone to allergies. There is also the possibility of phototoxicity when working with blends.

Regardless of these possible effects, essential oils are a viable option for supporting the body's defenses against a number of conditions. Those looking to enhance the maintenance of their own personal health, or that of their families, should become educated on the uses of essential oils, their natural remedies, and the methods of application. Only then can we begin building a kit of essential oils for survival.

Chapter 2:
Recipes for Cilantro Essential Oil

In this chapter, we will offer various recipes for Cilantro essential oil, both for pure Cilantro applications and blends. For pure supportive remedies, we have provided the appropriate application and dosage to support the body's natural function in addressing specific ailments, from ADD to metal detoxification. When it comes to blends, herbalists and aromatherapists often combine Cilantro essential oil with cinnamon, bergamot, grapefruit, orange, ginger, lime, lemon, neroli, and other citrus fruits oils. We will offer some fantastic supportive blending options in the second half of this chapter.

Pure Supportive Remedies

ADD/ADHD

Cilantro can help focus steady attention and concentration, particularly for those who suffer from attention deficit disorder. To apply, dilute Cilantro essential oil in a 1:1 ratio with a carrier oil and massage into the feet once a day; diffuse the oil throughout the room or inhale directly. Great for busy classrooms.

Anxiety

To relieve anxiety, place one drop of Cilantro essential oil into the palm and rub hands together. Place hand over nose and mouth and inhale; diffuse throughout home to alleviate tension and stress.

Cooking

Use Cilantro oil in cooking, as it is generally regarded as safe by the FDA. One drop (or less) to begin with; add more to taste. A little oil goes a long way.

Depression

Combat depression by placing a drop of Cilantro essential oil on pillow or in water or tea. Diffuse throughout the room, or dilute the oil in a 1:1 ratio with a carrier oil and apply topically, massaging into scalp, neck, and shoulders.

Detox

To support the body's systems through detoxification, combine Cilantro essential oil in a 1:1 ratio with a carrier oil and massage toward the heart, or apply 1 drop to a glass of drinking water and take internally.

Digestive Aid

Cilantro aids the digestive tract and can be taken orally or topically. Place a drop into drinking water for internal administration, or dilute the oil in a 1:1 ratio with a carrier oil and apply topically to the abdomen in a clockwise motion and into the reflex points of the feet. Diffuse throughout the home.

Heavy Metal Detox

To detoxify the body of heavy metals, combine Cilantro essential oil in a 1:1 ratio with a carrier oil and massage toward the heart. Apply 1 drop to a glass of drinking water and take internally.

Immune Stimulant

Give your immune system a leg up by regularly diffusing Cilantro throughout your home, especially during cold and flu season. The scent also uplifts and boosts energy. Alternatively, add a couple drops to bathwater or dilute in a 1:1 ratio with a carrier oil and apply topically, massaging the oil into the feet. Steam two drops of Cilantro essential oil in a pan of water, remove the steaming pan from the stove, pour into a bowl, place a towel over head and inhale.

Infection

To fight off infection, dilute Cilantro essential oil in a 1:1 ratio with a carrier oil and apply topically to the affected area, or to the soles of the feet. Diffuse throughout the room; whichever application is more appropriate to the specific condition.

Inflammation

Calm inflammation by diluting 1 or 2 drops of Cilantro essential oil in a 1:1 ratio with a carrier oil, then apply topically, massaging the oil over the affected area towards the heart.

Insomnia

With its calming and relaxing scent, Cilantro oil can help relieve insomnia. In order to trigger nervous system response, dilute in a 1:1 ratio with a carrier oil and apply topically to the reflex points in the feet. Diffuse or place a couple drops on pillow or sheets.

Lead Poisoning

Combat lead poisoning by combining Cilantro essential oil in a 1:1 ratio with a carrier oil and massaging toward the heart. Apply 1 drop to a glass of drinking water and take internally.

Muscular Support

Support muscular development by diluting Cilantro essential oil in a 1:1 ratio with a carrier oil and massaging the solution in a full-body massage, into the reflex points of the feet, or over the affected area. This application can also help with sports injuries, inflammation, strain, or soreness.

Stress

Combat stress by steaming two drops of Cilantro essential oil in a pan of water, remove the steaming pan from the stove, pour into a bowl, place a towel over head and inhale. Diffuse or place a drop onto shirt collar for portable stress relief.

Blends

Arthritic Pain Relief

Ingredients

1 drop Ginger Essential Oil

2 drops Cilantro Essential Oil

3 drops Cypress Essential Oil

2 Tbsps. Carrier Oil

Directions

Relieve arthritic pain by combining all ingredients in a small container. Tighten the lid and shake well. Apply topically, massaging into arthritic wrists or knees whenever in need of pain relief.

Circulation Stimulant

Ingredients

4 drops Cypress Essential Oil

2 drops Rosemary Essential Oil

2 drops Cilantro Essential Oil

2 drops Wild Orange Essential Oil

½ ounce Coconut Oil

Directions

To stimulate circulation, combine all ingredients in a small container, mixing until well blended. Apply topically to the ankles towards the heart.

Diabetes

Ingredients

2 drops Basil Essential Oil

3 drops Cilantro Essential Oil

1 tsp Carrier Oil

Directions

Apply topically to the reflex points in the feet and to the back of the neck and under the tongue two times a day.

Fatigue

Ingredients

1 drops Ginger Essential Oil

2 drops Clary Sage Essential Oil

2 drops Sandalwood Essential Oil

2 drops Cilantro Essential Oil

3 drops Frankincense Essential Oil

½ Tbsp. Carrier Oil

Directions

To combat fatigue, combine all ingredients in a small bowl or container, blending well. Apply topically to the forearms and the back of the neck, inhaling the scent deeply.

Liver Tonic Support

Ingredients

2 drops Patchouli Essential Oil

2 drops Marjoram Essential Oil

2 drops Bergamot Essential Oil

3 drops Frankincense Essential Oil

3 drops Cilantro Essential Oil

4 drops Cypress Essential Oil

1 tsp Carrier Oil

Directions

To support healthy liver function, combine all ingredients in a small container and mix well. Every evening for up to two weeks, apply topically the area of the liver (right side of the body, below the ribs) and to the soles of the feet.

Lymphatic Salve

Ingredients

4 drops Cypress Essential Oil

3 drops Cilantro Essential Oil

3 drops Lime Essential Oil

3 drops White Fir Essential Oil

2 drops Patchouli Essential Oil

2 drops Rosemary Essential Oil

3 Tbsps. Coconut Oil

Directions

To relieve leg or feet swelling or edema due to hot/humid weather, combine all ingredients in a small bowl or glass container and mix well. Apply topically for three days, once in the morning and once in the evening, to the outside of the leg, from the knee up to above the waist.

Odor Eliminator

Ingredients

1 drop Melaleuca Essential Oil

1 drop White Fir Essential Oil

1 drop Cilantro Essential Oil

1 drop Lime Essential Oil

2 drops Lemon Essential Oil

Directions

To eliminate odors throughout home, diffuse this blend. Great for animal lovers.

Upset Stomach

Ingredients

1 drop Rosemary Essential Oil

1 drop Cilantro Essential Oil

½ glass Warm Drinking Water

Directions

To alleviate upset stomach, combine rosemary and Cilantro in drinking water. Stir well and drink.

Chapter 3:
Cilantro Essential Oil Studies

Many studies have been done on essential oils to uncover and prove their therapeutic qualities. In the case of the great number of Cilantro studies, many of the properties attributed to the essential oil (noted in this book and elsewhere) are quite often validated through the research from accredited universities and published by reputable scientific journals. In this chapter, we will discuss a small portion of these studies. It is important to note that research on essential oils is constant and evolving. Keep up with any recent research, as it may turn up even further valuable uses of these miracle oils.

Study 1 – Liver Support

In this study published by the *Journal of Pharmacy & BioAllied Sciences,* the effects of Cilantro essential oil on the liver were examined, with the following results: "Coriandrum sativum (Linn.), a glabrous, aromatic, herbaceous annual plant, is well known for its use in jaundice. Essential oil, flavonoids, fatty acids, and sterols have been isolated from different parts of C. sativum…The results of this study have led to the conclusion that ethanolic extract of C. sativum possesses hepatoprotective activity which may be due to the antioxidant potential of phenolic compounds."

Hepatotoxicity means liver damage, which is why hepatoprotection relates to the ability to protect against liver damage. The study revealed that essential oil from the Cilantro was high in antioxidants and showed activity against carbon tetrachloride, a chemical found in everything from pesticides and fire extinguishers to refrigerants and cleaning agents. Carbon tetrachloride is often used in research to identify hepatoprotective agents, as it is amongst the most potent hepatotoxins.

Cilantro essential oil helped to reduce the liver weight and the carbon tetrachloride activity in the animals tested. In fact, a 300 mg/kg dose of C. sativum extract completely eliminated the fatty deposit, the degeneration and necrosis (premature death of cells), which demonstrated the oil's antihepatotoxic activity, suggesting that Cilantro is an effective liver support.

Reference:
http://www.ncbi.nlm.nih.gov/pubmed/21966166]

http://www.ncbi.nlm.nih.gov/pmc/articles/PMC3178952/

Study 2 – Antifungal Properties

In this study published by the journal, *Molecules*, the antifungal effects of Cilantro essential were examined, with the following results: "The aims of this study were to test the antifungal activity, toxicity and chemical composition of essential oil from C. sativum L. fruits. The essential oil, obtained by hydrodistillation, was analyzed by gas chromatography/mass spectroscopy...C. sativum essential oil is active in vitro against M. canis and Candida spp. demonstrating good antifungal activity."

The study tested Cilantro essential oil against several Candida strains, as well as Microsporum canis. Microsporum canis is a fungus that can cause ringworm in animals and tinea capitis in humans. Tinea capitis is a superficial fungal infection of the scalp that can sometimes include scaling, itching, inflammation, and pustules. Several Candida species were tested, including Candida albicans, which develops as yeast and filamentous cells, and can potentially cause genital and oral infections. Candida albicans also increases the probability of mortality in immunocompromised individuals (cancer or AIDS patients, for instance).

The essential oil of Cilantro leaves was also tested against Escherichia coli and Salmonella typhi. E. coli is a Gram-negative bacterium that can often result in serious food poisoning. Salmonella strains can cause an array of illnesses from typhoid fever to food poisoning.

Cilantro essential oil showed good antifungal and antibacterial activity against all strains of fungi and bacteria tested, which demonstrates that the oil can support a wide range of infections.

Reference:
http://www.ncbi.nlm.nih.gov/pubmed/22785271

http://www.mdpi.com/1420-3049/17/7/8439]

Study 3 – Oral Hygiene

In this study published by *PLOS*, the effects of Cilantro essential oil on oral hygiene were examined, with the following results: "Oral candidiasis is an opportunistic fungal infection of the oral cavity with increasingly worldwide prevalence and incidence rates. Novel specifically-targeted strategies to manage this ailment have been proposed using essential oils (EO) known to have antifungal properties. In this study, we aim to investigate the antifungal activity and mode of action of the EO from Coriandrum sativum L. (coriander) leaves on Candida spp…the findings highlight the potential antifungal activity of the EO from C. sativum leaves and suggest avenues for future translational toxicological research."

As noted, the study examined the effects of Cilantro essential oil on oral pathogens, produced by fungi from the Candida species. Candida albicans develops as yeast and filamentous cells and can potentially cause genital and oral infections.

This study found that the minimum inhibitory concentration (MIC) and the minimum fungicidal concentration (MFC) of Cilantro essential oil was exceptionally effective against this strain of fungi, indicating that Cilantro essential oil can be used as an oral antifungal against these pathogens and many more.

Reference:
http://www.ncbi.nlm.nih.gov/pubmed/24901768

http://www.ncbi.nlm.nih.gov/pmc/articles/PMC4047076/
pdf/pone.0099086.pdf]

Study 4 – Alzheimer's Disease

In this study available on PubMed, the effects of Cilantro essential oil on anxiety and depression in those suffering from Alzheimer's Disease were examined, with the following results: "The present study analyzed the possible anxiolytic, antidepressant and antioxidant properties of inhaled coriander (or Cilantro) volatile oil extracted from Coriandrum sativum var. microcarpum in beta-amyloid (1-42) rat model of Alzheimer's disease...Exposure to coriander volatile oil significantly improved these parameters, suggesting anxiolytic- and antidepressant-like effects. Moreover, coriander volatile oil decreased catalase activity and increased glutathione level in the hippocampus. Our results suggest that multiple exposures to coriander volatile oil can be useful as a mean to counteract anxiety, depression and oxidative stress in Alzheimer's disease conditions."

This study took a look at the anxiolytic, antidepressant and antioxidant effect of Cilantro essential oil on rats with beta-amyloid (1-42), a model of Alzheimer's disease. The rats were then subjected to forced swimming tests and elevated plus-mazes in order to test the anxiolytic effects. The antioxidant activity was also assessed within the hippocampus, the area of the brain that is particularly significant when it comes to stress, as this is the area that processes prior memories, which then suppress or enhance a stress response. After application of Cilantro essential oil, the rats' locomotor activity and times during the swimming and maze tests greatly improved. This demonstrates that Cilantro may be effective in combating oxidative stress, anxiety or depression in relation to Alzheimer's.

Reference
http://www.ncbi.nlm.nih.gov/pubmed/24747275]

Study 5 – Antioxidant & Anticancer Properties

In this study published by *BMC Complementary & Alternative Medicine*, the antioxidant and anticancer effects of Cilantro essential oil were examined, with the following results: "Coriandrum sativum is a popular culinary and medicinal herb of the Apiaceae family. Health promoting properties of this herb have been reported in pharmacognostical, phytochemical and pharmacological studies. However, studies on C. sativum have always focused on the aerial parts of the herb and scientific investigation on the root is limited. The aim of this research was to investigate the antioxidant and anticancer activities of C. sativum root, leaf and stem, including its effect on cancer cell migration, and its protection against DNA damage, with special focus on the roots…This study is the first report on the antioxidant and anticancer properties of C. sativum root. The herb shows potential in preventing oxidative stress-related diseases and would be useful as supplements used in combination with conventional drugs to enhance the treatment of diseases such as cancer."

This study analyzed the effects of Cilantro essential oil on MCF-7 cells. MCF-7 is a breast cancer cell line. When the cell line is broached by Cilantro essential oil, the result is cell death. In multicellular organisms, apoptosis is the process of programmed cell death. In the case of cancer, an insufficient amount of apoptosis results in an unmanageable growth of cancer cells, so the cell death stimulated by

Cilantro essential oil is necessary to control the cancer. Cilantro essential oil was also shown to possess high antioxidant activity, which demonstrates that the oil can be used in supporting the body's defenses against oxidative stress.

Reference:
http://www.ncbi.nlm.nih.gov/pubmed/24517259]

http://www.ncbi.nlm.nih.gov/pmc/articles/PMC4028854/pdf/1472-6882-13-347.pdf]

Study 6 – Diabetes

In this study available on PubMed, the effects of Cilantro essential oil on diabetes were examined, with the following results: "In India's indigenous system of medicine, Coriandrum sativum (CS), commonly used as a food ingredient, is claimed to be useful for various ailments. To establish its utility in diabetes mellitus, the present study evaluated the antidiabetic and antioxidant effects of CS in alloxan-induced diabetic rats…These results indicate that the extracts could protect liver function and exhibited hypoglycemic, hypolipidemic, and antioxidant efficacies in the diabetic rats. These results support the use of this plant extract to manage diabetes mellitus."

This study was a comparative analysis of the effects of Cilantro essential oil against those of the diabetic clinical drug, glibenclamide. The effectiveness of the two substances was measured by the blood glucose, total cholesterol, triglycerides, and low-density lipoprotein cholesterol levels in diabetic rats. Cilantro essential oil demonstrated high antioxidant levels, with free radical scavenging effects comparable to the reference antioxidants. Moreover, the oil's antioxidant potential increased through catalyzing enzymes and reducing lipid peroxidation, which refers to a process in which electrons are "stolen" by free radicals from lipids, causing cell damage and the oxidative degradation of lipids. These results indicated that Cilantro essential oil can, in fact, be applied to diabetic maintenance, as well as to support liver function.

Reference
http://www.ncbi.nlm.nih.gov/pubmed/22671941]

Chapter 4:
The Ins & Outs of Essential Oils

Where do essential oils come from?

Plants and plant species naturally produce essential oils for various reasons, one being to draw pollinator insects to them, another being to repel invading organisms (bacteria, animals). A number of chemical compounds compose each plant's essential oil, and the combination of these compounds are specific to each oil, which then instills in the oil its own unique properties. Essential oils can be harnessed from all sorts of plant components, including flowers, leaves, bark, fruit, roots, and resin. For instance, cinnamon oil is harnessed from bark, lemon oil from the peel, and lavender oil from flowers. Certain plants can produce a few chemical variants of the same essential oil, which are acquired from different parts of the plant. Some of these parts produce a large amount of oil, while others produce just a smidgen. The oil's quality and potency depends upon a number of factors, including the subspecies of the plant, its soil conditions, the time of year and even the time of day it is harvested.

How are essential oils extracted?

Essential oils can be extracted from plants through various methods, including pressing, distillation, solvent and maceration. Let's take a brief look at each:

Pressing Method

Commonly used with citrus fruit, the pressing method extracts the oil through a technique which involves pushing the fruit peels through a press. Oily fruits and plants are best suited for this technique. Orange oil, for example, is extracted from orange skins through the pressing method.

Distillation Method

This technique harkens back to the days of moonshiners, as the same sort of method used to create strong liquor can be used to extract essential oils. Using a still, boiled water and plant materials will create steam which is then cooled by coils and condensed into a combination of water and oil. This combination does not mix, so the oil can then be extracted from it.

Solvent Method

Through a multi-step process, certain plant and flower oils can be extracted using alcohol and other solvents, which extort the essential oil from the plant materials.

Maceration Method

When a "carrier," fixed oil, or lard is mixed with the plant material and set out in the sun, over a period of time, the carrier oil is infused with the plant's essence. Heat sources, other than the sun, are often used to speed the process. Throughout the process, more plant material is added to produce a more potent oil.

How do you use essential oils?

Although some studies about the effectiveness of essential oils are conducted by small companies or even individuals, a number of them are conducted by the food and cosmetic industries. In general, the pharmaceutical industry shows next to no interest in herbal medicine, primarily because there are few options to patent such products. As such, the product's lack of profitability results in a lack of research funding. Regardless, the historical uses of essential oils tell us what we need to know: these oils have been effectively administered for centuries. The therapeutic qualifications of essential oils can be plotted in the survival of the human race across cultures and generations.

Another reason that studies on essential oils have not resulted in much conclusive evidence as to their overall effectiveness is because definitive results are sometimes difficult to prove, as the quality of each batch of oil can vary for a number of reasons. One is that essential oils are impossible to standardize. As mentioned above, even the slightest variance in soil conditions and the time of harvesting – as well as innumerable other factors – will produce a different product quality and potency. In addition, essential oils are often obtained from various species of the same plant; Eucalyptus radiata and Eucalyptus globulus can both be used in the making of therapeutic-grade eucalyptus oil and as a result, they may have slightly different properties and degrees of strength or effectiveness.

Just as there are a number of methods by which to extract essential oils, there are a number of methods to administer them therapeutically. The variety of chemical compounds in each essential oil means that their benefits and applications also vary across the board. Below are a few of these methods.

Topical Administration

Direct application of many essential oils works like a sponge, as skin absorbs chemicals and other things (like sunlight, for instance). Topical application is best when you want to clear up an ailment on the skin's surface, or in the underlying muscle tissue. When applying topically, either massage the oil into the skin, or simply dab on the skin for therapeutic results. Combine the essential oil with a carrier oil for topical use in order to dilute its potency. This is safer, as the oil is very concentrated. Support the body's defenses against rash or muscle pain in this manner, but you should always test a patient for allergies before applying. Adverse effects are produced by natural chemicals as much as synthetic ones; poison ivy, for example.

To test for allergens, place a drop or two on your patient's inner forearm. If a rash develops within 12 to 24 hours, then the patient is allergic. In addition, phototoxicity – sun exposure resulting in an exacerbated burn – may be an issue when citrus oils are applied topically. One must proceed with caution when applying essential oils using this method.

Inhalation Therapy

Commonly known as "aromatherapy," this essential oil application is effective for inner ailments, like sore throat or cold. In a steaming bowl of distilled or sterilized water, add a few drops of essential oil and with a towel over the head, bend over the bowl and inhale. The towel captures the vapors, making the technique even more effective. Essential oils can also be placed in a diffuser, or potpourri, throughout a room to produce somewhat diluted medicinal effects.

Ingestion

When using this method proceed with caution. Direct ingestion of essential oils must be monitored and applied in small doses that are diluted in a tablespoon or more of any carrier oil – olive oil, for example. If unsure of dosage amounts, make a tea with the relevant herb instead. Although the effects of this diluted use may be weaker, this application is a better alternative than an overdose of essential oils.

What are the general benefits of using essential oils?

Replacement for Prescription Drugs

One practical benefit for using essential oils is of course, their substitutive nature; they can replace Rx drugs, which is the ultimate reason to educate yourself on their administration and to begin stockpiling an essential oil supply. One of the potential threats of economic, or social collapse, is the lack of resources, and primarily the inability to procure prescription drugs. As such, finding suitable alternatives should be a priority when prepping for the worst.

Their portability is also a major bonus when it comes to survival prepping. The fact that these ultra-concentrated oils take up little-to-no space makes toting them to a shelter all the simpler should the need arise. Because essential oils are highly concentrated, the application used in most methods of administration requires only a drop or two of oil, which means that a tiny bottle will be long-lasting.

Cost Efficient, yet Effective Alternative

Though money may be the last thing on your mind when it comes to prepping for a survival situation (money may even be obsolete in the event of social collapse), it is worth noting that the expense of essential oils pales in comparison to prescription drugs. In fact, whether or not you are forced to survive on essential oils due to a lack of prescription reserves, in some cases, you might consider substituting prescriptions for these inexpensive alternatives regardless. Essential oils are a cost effective, but equally effective alternative to prescription medicine.

No Expiration Date

Another benefit of essential oils is that they do not expire, nor do they have "proper storage" requirements. A number of medicines and medicinal products must be replaced every couple of years; this sets essential oils ahead of the pack when it comes to shelf life.

Versatility

Essential oils also offer great versatility. Apart from providing health benefits, essential oils can be repurposed for household and hygienic applications. For instance, if looking for something that might serve dental hygiene needs in a time of crisis, thieves oil is the go-to essential oil. In order to maintain the skin's health, frankincense and lavender will do the trick; the latter also serves as sunscreen, so it can protect against sun damage as well.

When it comes to the house or shelter, use essential

oils to deodorize, which will come in handy in a disaster scenario where things might start to smell bad due to lack of proper utilities and care. For example, after the 2011 tsunami and the subsequent nuclear reactor meltdown in Japan, a nurse named Risa Nakahira used essential oils to deodorize and sanitize putrid public bathrooms in overpopulated evacuation facilities. As relief workers searched for survivors, often wading through debris and decay, Nakahira also deodorized their boots and masks using essential oils. The possibilities of these natural oils are endless.

They are also versatile when it comes to the range of patients they are capable of supporting. The health of everyone from great grandfather to infant baby can be fortified with the aid of essential oils in the appropriate dosage. They even come in handy when supporting the health of livestock or pets. From teething infants to dementia in the elderly, from teenagers with acne to dogs with urinary tract infections, essential oils can serve any patient with nearly any ailment.

Conclusion

Now that you know all about what Cilantro essential oil can do for you – where it originates, how it is extracted, its benefits and properties, and the different methods of administration – you can use it confidently to support the body's defenses against health issues and start to assemble a kit of essential oils for survival. Essential oils can be purchased online or at your local holistic treatment store.

The various benefits of essential oils and their properties are countless. To build your own kit, first focus on acquiring the essential oils which may bear more relevance to specific health issues, or the potential health threats within the environment. In the event of a heavy metal detoxification, for instance, Cilantro essential oil will be one of your more crucial oils, due to its supportive properties.

Used as a supplement or as your go-to for muscular and digestive support, psychological health, or infections, the application of Cilantro essential oil in medicine has survived for centuries and will survive centuries more. When it comes down to it, you do not need to rely on pharmaceuticals; essential oils, herbs, and plenty of other natural ingredients can be used to help support any number of health issues, whether ailment or injury.

Essential oils are essential to your survival in the case of viral outbreak, social collapse or natural disaster because, when the SHTF, your access to pharmaceuticals will likely be limited or eliminated altogether. Alternatives to our modern-day standard will equate survival when no other option exists. And when it comes to a life-or-death situation, you cannot let your health decline, no matter the state of the world..

DISCLAIMER AND/OR LEGAL NOTICES: Every effort has been made to accurately represent this book and it's potential. Results vary with every individual, and your results may or may not be different from those depicted. No promises, guarantees or warranties, whether stated or implied, have been made that you will produce any specific result from this book. Your efforts are individual and unique, and may vary from those shown. Your success depends on your efforts, background and motivation.

The material in this publication is provided for educational and informational purposes only and is not intended as medical advice. The information contained in this book should not be used to diagnose or treat any illness, metabolic disorder, disease or health problem. Always consult your physician or healthcare provider before beginning any nutrition or exercise program. Use of the programs, advice, and information contained in this book is at the sole choice and risk of the reader.